MW01230972

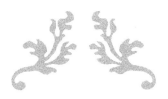

Mastering Wood Pellet Smoker And Grill

A Step-By-Step Guide To Become An Expert Barbecue Pitmaster
With Your Grill With Recipes For The Best-Of Smoking & Bbq

LIAM JONES

by any usage or abuse of any policies, processes, or Instructions contained within is the solitary and utter responsibility of the recipient reader. Under no circumstances will any legal responsibility or blame be held against the publisher for any reparation, damages, or monetary loss due to the information herein, either directly or indirectly.

The information herein is offered for informational purposes solely and is universal as such. The presentation of the information is without a contract or any type of guarantee assurance.

The trademarks that are used are without any consent and the publication of the trademark is without permission or backing by the trademark owner. All trademarks and brands within this book are for clarifying purposes only and are owned by the owners themselves, not affiliated with this document.

Table of Contents

BREAKFAST RECIPES

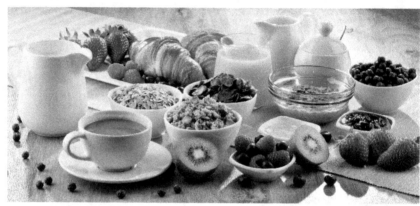

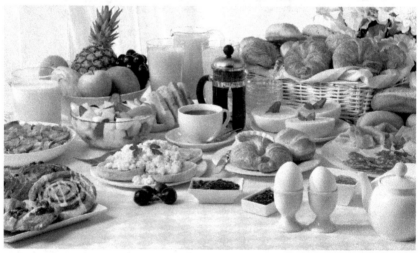

1. *Spicy Sausage & Cheese Balls*

Preparation Time: 20 minutes

Cooking Time: 40 minutes

Servings: 4

Ingredients:

- 1lb Hot Breakfast Sausage
- 2 cups Bisquick Baking Mix
- 8 ounces Cream Cheese
- 8 ounces Extra Sharp Cheddar Cheese
- 1/4 cup Fresno Peppers
- 1 tablespoon Dried Parsley
- 1 teaspoon Killer Hogs AP Rub
- 1/2 teaspoon Onion Powder

Directions:

1. Get ready smoker or flame broil for roundabout cooking at 400 degrees F.
2. Blend Sausage, Baking Mix, destroyed cheddar, cream cheddar, and remaining fixings in a huge bowl until all-around fused.
3. Utilize a little scoop to parcel blend into chomp to estimate balls and roll tenderly fit as a fiddle.

4. Spot wiener and cheddar balls on a cast-iron container and cook for 15mins.

5. Present with your most loved plunging sauces.

Nutrition: Calories: 95 Carbs: 4g Fat: 7g Protein: 5g

2. White Chocolate Bread Pudding

Preparation Time: 20 minutes

Cooking Time: 1hr 15 minutes

Servings: 12

Ingredients:

- 1 loaf of French bread
- 4 cups Heavy Cream
- 3 Large Eggs
- 2 cups White Sugar
- 1 package White Chocolate morsels
- ¼ cup Melted Butter
- 2 teaspoons Vanilla
- 1 teaspoon Ground Nutmeg
- 1 teaspoon Salt
- Bourbon White Chocolate Sauce
- 1 package White Chocolate morsels
- 1 cup Heavy Cream
- 2 tablespoons Melted Butter
- 2 tablespoons Bourbon
- ½ teaspoon Salt

Directions:

1. Get ready pellet smoker or any flame broil/smoker for backhanded cooking at 350 degrees F.

2. Tear French bread into little portions and spot it in a massive bowl. Pour four cups of Heavy Cream over Bread and douse for 30mins.

3. Join eggs, sugar, softened spread, and vanilla in a medium to estimate bowl. Include a package of white chocolate pieces and a delicate blend. Season with Nutmeg and Salt.

4. Pour egg combo over the splashed French bread and blend to sign up for.

5. Pour the combination right into a properly to buttered nine X 13 to inchmeal dish and spot it at the smoker.

6. Cook for 60Secs or until bread pudding has set and the top is darker.

7. For the sauce: Melt margarine in a saucepot over medium warm temperature. Add whiskey and hold on cooking for three to 4mins until liquor vanished and margarine begins to darkish-colored.

8. Include vast cream and heat till a mild stew. Take from the warmth and consist of white chocolate pieces a bit at a time continuously blending until the complete percent has softened. Season with a hint of salt and serve over bread pudding.

Nutrition: Calories: 372 Carbs: 31g Fat: 25g Protein: 5g

3. *Cheesy Jalapeño Skillet Dip*

Preparation Time: 10 minutes

Cooking Time: 15 minutes

Servings: 8

Ingredients:

- 8 ounces cream cheese
- 16 ounces shredded cheese
- 1/3 cup mayonnaise
- 4 ounces diced green chilies
- 3 fresh jalapeños
- 2 teaspoons Killer Hogs AP Rub
- 2 teaspoons Mexican Style Seasoning

For the topping:

- ¼ cup Mexican Blend Shredded Cheese
- Sliced jalapeños
- Mexican Style Seasoning
- 3 tablespoons Killer Hogs AP Rub
- 2 tablespoons Chili Powder
- 2 tablespoons Paprika
- 2 teaspoons Cumin
- ½ teaspoon Granulated Onion
- ¼ teaspoon Cayenne Pepper

- ¼ teaspoon Chipotle Chili Pepper ground
- ¼ teaspoon Oregano

Directions:

1. Preheat smoker or flame broil for roundabout cooking at 350 degree
2. Join fixings in a big bowl and spot in a cast to press skillet
3. Top with Mexican Blend destroyed cheddar and cuts of jalapeno's
4. Spot iron skillet on flame broil mesh and cook until cheddar hot and bubbly and the top has seared
5. Marginally about 25mins.
6. Serve warm with enormous corn chips (scoops), tortilla chips, or your preferred vegetables for plunging.

Nutrition: Calories: 150 Carbs: 22g Fat: 6g Protein: 3g

4. *Cajun Turkey Club*

Preparation Time: 5 Minutes

Cooking Time: 10 Minutes

Servings: 3

Ingredients:

- 1 3lbs Turkey Breast
- 1 stick Butter (melted)
- 8 ounces Chicken Broth
- 1 tablespoon Killer Hogs Hot Sauce
- 1/4 cup Malcolm's King Craw Seasoning
- 8 Pieces to Thick Sliced Bacon
- 1 cup Brown Sugar
- 1 head Green Leaf Lettuce
- 1 Tomato (sliced)
- 6 slices Toasted Bread
- ½ cup Cajun Mayo
- 1 cup Mayo
- 1 tablespoon Dijon Mustard
- 1 tablespoon Killer Hogs Sweet Fire Pickles (chopped)
- 1 tablespoon Horseradish
- ½ teaspoon Malcolm's King Craw Seasoning
- 1 teaspoon Killer Hogs Hot Sauce

- Pinch of Salt & Black Pepper to taste

Directions:

1. Get ready pellet smoker for backhanded cooking at 325 degrees F utilizing your preferred wood pellets for enhancing.

2. Join dissolved margarine, chicken stock, hot sauce, and 1 tbsp of Cajun Seasoning in a blending bowl. Infuse the blend into the turkey bosom scattering the infusion destinations for even inclusion.

3. Shower the outside of the turkey bosom with a Vegetable cooking splash and season with Malcolm's King Craw Seasoning.

4. Spot the turkey bosom on the smoker and cook until the inside temperature arrives at 165 degrees. Utilize a moment-read thermometer to screen temp during the cooking procedure.

5. Consolidate darker sugar and 1 teaspoon of King Craw in a little bowl. Spread the bacon with the sugar blend and spot it on a cooling rack.

6. Cook the bacon for 12 to 15mins or until darker. Make certain to turn the bacon part of the way through for cooking.

7. Toast the bread, cut the tomatoes dainty, and wash/dry the lettuce leaves.

8. At the point when the turkey bosom arrives at 165 take it from the flame broil and rest for 15mins. Take the netting out from around the bosom and cut into slender cuts.

9. To cause the sandwich: To slather Cajun Mayo* on the toast, stack on a few cuts of turkey bosom, lettuce, tomato, and bacon. Include another bit of toast and rehash a similar procedure. Include the top bit of toast slathered with more Cajun mayo, cut the sandwich into equal parts and appreciate.

Nutrition: Calories: 130 Carbs: 1g Fat: 4g Protein: 21g

FISH AND SEAFOOD RECIPES

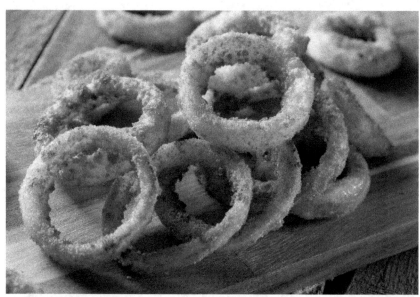

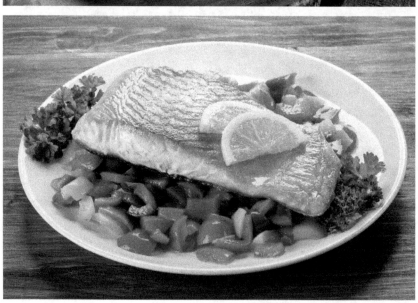

5. Grilled King Crab Legs

Preparation Time: 10 minutes

Cooking Time: 25 minutes

Servings: 4

Ingredients:

- 4 pounds king crab legs (split)
- 4 tbsp. lemon juice
- 2 tbsp. garlic powder
- 1 cup butter (melted)
- 2 tsp. brown sugar
- 2 tsp. paprika
- 2 tsp. ground black pepper or more to taste

Directions:

1. In a mixing bowl, combine the lemon juice, butter, sugar, garlic, paprika, and pepper.
2. Arrange the split crab on a baking sheet, split side up.
3. Drizzle ¾ of the butter mixture over the crab legs.
4. Configure your pellet grill for indirect cooking and preheat it to 225°F, using mesquite wood pellets.
5. Arrange the crab legs onto the grill grate, shell side down.
6. Cover the grill and cook for 25 minutes.
7. Remove the crab legs from the grill.
8. Serve and top with the remaining butter mixture.

Nutrition: Amount per 371 g = 1 serving(s) Energy (calories): 513 kcal Protein: 12.94 g Fat: 33.65 g Carbohydrates: 42.19 g

6. *Togarashi Smoked Salmon*

Preparation Time: 20 hours

Cooking Time: 4 hours

Servings: 10

Ingredients:

- 2 large salmon filet
- Togarashi for seasoning

For Brine:

- 1 cup brown sugar
- 4 cups of water
- 1/3 cup kosher salt

Directions:

1. Remove all the thorns from the fish filet.
2. Mix all the brine ingredients until the brown sugar is dissolved completely.
3. Put the mix in a big bowl and add the filet to it.
4. Leave the bowl to refrigerate for 16 hours.
5. After 16 hours, remove the salmon from this mix. Wash and dry it.
6. Place the salmon in the refrigerator for another 2-4 hours. (This step is essential. DO NOT SKIP IT.)
7. Season your salmon filet with Togarashi.

8. Start the wood pellet grill with the 'smoke' option and place the salmon on it.

9. Smoke for 4 hours.

10. Make sure the temperature does not go above 180 degrees or below 130 degrees.

11. Remove from the grill and serve it warm with a side dish of your choice.

Nutrition: Amount per 68 g = 1 serving(s) Energy (calories): 57 kcal Protein: 6.55 g Fat: 1.23 g Carbohydrates: 4.99 g

7. *Grilled Shrimp*

Preparation Time:

Cooking Time: 15 minutes

Servings: 4

Ingredients:

- 1 lb. jumbo shrimp peeled and cleaned
- 2 tbsp. oil
- ½ tbsp. salt
- 4-5 skewers
- 1/8 tbsp. pepper
- ½ tbsp. garlic salt

Directions:

1. Preheat the wood pellet grill to 375 degrees.
2. Mix all the ingredients in a small bowl.
3. After washing and drying the shrimp, mix it well with the oil and seasonings.
4. Add skewers to the shrimp and set the bowl of shrimp aside.
5. Open the skewers and flip them.
6. Cook for four more minutes. Remove when the shrimp is opaque and pink.

Nutrition: Amount per 63 g = 1 serving(s) Energy (calories): 88 kcal Protein: 11.63 g Fat: 4.18 g Carbohydrates: 0.25 g

CHICKEN AND TURKEY RECIPES

8. Smoked Turkey Breast

Preparation Time: 10 Minutes

Cooking Time: 1 Hour 30 minutes

Servings: 6

Ingredients:

- For The Brine
- 1 Cup of kosher salt
- 1 Cup of maple syrup
- ¼ Cup of brown sugar
- ¼ Cup of whole black peppercorns
- 4 Cups of cold bourbon
- 1 and ½ gallons of cold water
- 1 Turkey breast of about 7 pounds

For Turkey

- 3 Tablespoons of brown sugar
- 1 and ½ tablespoons of smoked paprika
- 1 ½ teaspoon of chipotle chili powder
- 1 ½ teaspoon of garlic powder
- 1 ½ teaspoon of salt

- 1 and ½ teaspoons of black pepper
- 1 teaspoon of onion powder
- ½ teaspoon of ground cumin
- 6 Tablespoons of melted unsalted butter

Directions:

1. Before beginning; make sure that the bourbon; the water and the chicken stock are all cold

2. Now to make the brine, combine altogether the salt, the syrup, the sugar, the peppercorns, the bourbon, and the water in a large bucket.

3. Remove any pieces that are left on the turkey, like the neck or the giblets

4. Refrigerate the turkey meat in the brine for about 8 to 12 hours in a resealable bag

5. Remove the turkey breast from the brine and pat dry with clean paper towels; then place it over a baking sheet and refrigerate for about 1 hour

6. Preheat your pellet smoker to about 300°F; making sure to add the wood chips to the burner

7. In a bowl, mix the paprika with the sugar, the chili powder, the garlic powder, the salt, the pepper, the onion powder, and the cumin, mixing very well to combine.

8. Carefully lift the skin of the turkey; then rub the melted butter over the meat

9. Rub the spice over the meat very well and over the skin

10. Smoke the turkey breast for about 1 ½ hour at a temperature of about 375°

Nutrition: Calories: 94 Fat: 2g Carbs: 1g Protein: 18g

9. *Herbed Turkey Breast*

Preparation Time: 8 Hours And 10 Minutes

Cooking Time: 3 Hours

Servings: 12

Ingredients:

- 7 pounds turkey breast, bone-in, skin-on, fat trimmed
- 3/4 cup salt
- 1/3 cup brown sugar
- 4 quarts water, cold
- For Herbed Butter:
- 1 tablespoon chopped parsley
- ½ teaspoon ground black pepper
- 8 tablespoons butter, unsalted, softened
- 1 tablespoon chopped sage
- ½ tablespoon minced garlic
- 1 tablespoon chopped rosemary
- 1 teaspoon lemon zest
- 1 tablespoon chopped oregano
- 1 tablespoon lemon juice

Directions:

1. Prepare the brine and for this, pour water in a large container, add salt and sugar and stir well until salt and sugar have completely dissolved.

2. Add turkey breast in the brine, cover with the lid and let soak in the refrigerator for a minimum of 8 hours.

3. Then remove turkey breast from the brine, rinse well and pat dry with paper towels.

4. Open the hopper of the smoker, add dry pallets, make sure ash-can is in place, then open the ash damper, power on the smoker, and close the ash damper.

5. Set the temperature of the smoker to 350 degrees F, let preheat for 30 minutes or until the green light on the dial blinks that indicate the smoker has reached to set temperature.

6. Meanwhile, take a roasting pan, pour in 1 cup water, then place a wire rack in it and place turkey breast on it.

7. Prepare the herb butter and for this, place butter in a heatproof bowl, add remaining ingredients for the butter and stir until just mix.

8. Loosen the skin of the turkey from its breast by using your fingers, then insert 2 tablespoons of prepared herb butter on each side of the skin of the breastbone and spread it evenly, pushing out all the air pockets.

9. Place the remaining herb butter in the bowl into the microwave wave and heat for 1 minute or more at a high heat setting or until melted.

10. Then brush melted herb butter on the outside of the turkey breast and place roasting pan containing turkey on the smoker grill.

11. Shut the smoker with lid and smoke for 2 hours and 30 minutes or until the turkey breast is nicely golden brown and the internal temperature of turkey reach 165 degrees F, flipping the turkey and basting with melted herb butter after 1 hour and 30 minutes smoking.

12. When done, transfer the turkey breast to a cutting board, let it rest for 15 minutes, then carve it into pieces and serve.

Nutrition: Calories: 97 Fat: 4 g Protein: 13 g Carbs: 1 g

10. Jalapeno Injection Turkey

Preparation Time: 15 Minutes

Cooking Time: 4 Hours And 10 Minutes

Servings: 4

Ingredients:

- 15 pounds whole turkey, giblet removed
- ½ of medium red onion, peeled and minced
- 8 jalapeño peppers
- 2 tablespoons minced garlic
- 4 tablespoons garlic powder
- 6 tablespoons Italian seasoning
- 1 cup butter, softened, unsalted
- ¼ cup olive oil
- 1 cup chicken broth

Directions:

1. Open the hopper of the smoker, add dry pallets, make sure ash-can is in place, then open the ash damper, power on the smoker, and close the ash damper.

2. Make the temperature of the smoker up to 200 degrees F, let preheat for 30 minutes or until the green light on the dial blinks that indicate the smoker has reached to set temperature.

3. Meanwhile, place a large saucepan over medium-high heat, add oil and butter and when the butter melts, add onion, garlic, and peppers and cook for 3 to 5 minutes or until nicely golden brown.

4. Pour in broth, stir well, let the mixture boil for 5 minutes, then remove the pan from the heat and strain the mixture to get just liquid.

5. Inject turkey generously with prepared liquid, then spray the outside of turkey with butter spray and season well with garlic and Italian seasoning.

6. Place turkey on the smoker grill, shut with lid, and smoke for 30 minutes, then increase the temperature to 325 degrees F and continue smoking the turkey for 3 hours or until the internal temperature of turkey reach 165 degrees F.

7. When done, transfer turkey to a cutting board, let rest for 5 minutes, then carve into slices and serve.

Nutrition: Calories: 131 Fat: 7 g Protein: 13 g Carbs: 3 g

11. *Buttery Smoked Turkey Beer*

Preparation Time: 15 minutes

Cooking Time: 4 hours

Servings: 6

Ingredients:

- Whole turkey (4-lbs., 1.8-kg.)
- The Brine
- Beer – 2 cans
- Salt – 1 tablespoon
- White sugar – 2 tablespoons
- Soy sauce – ¼ cup
- Coldwater – 1 quart
- The Rub
- Unsalted butter – 3 tablespoons
- Smoked paprika – 1 teaspoon
- Garlic powder – 1 ½ teaspoon
- Pepper – 1 teaspoon
- Cayenne pepper – ¼ teaspoon

Directions:

1. Pour beer into a container then add salt, white sugar, and soy sauce then stir well.

2. Put the turkey into the brine mixture cold water over the turkey. Make sure that the turkey is completely soaked.

3. Soak the turkey in the brine for at least 6 hours or overnight and store it in the fridge to keep it fresh.

4. On the next day, remove the turkey from the fridge and take it out of the brine mixture.

5. Wash and rinse the turkey then pat it dry.

6. Next, plug the wood pellet smoker then fill the hopper with the wood pellet. Turn the switch on.

7. Set the wood pellet smoker for indirect heat then adjust the temperature to 275°F (135°C).

8. Open the beer can then push it into the turkey cavity.

9. Place the seasoned turkey in the wood pellet smoker and make a tripod using the beer can and the two turkey legs.

10. Smoke the turkey for 4 hours or until the internal temperature has reached 170°F (77°C).

11. Once it is done, remove the smoked turkey from the wood pellet smoker and transfer it to a serving dish.

Nutrition: Calories: 229 Carbs: 34g Fat: 8g Protein: 3g

12. Sweet Smoked Chicken in Black Tea Aroma

Preparation Time: 30 minutes

Cooking Time: 10 Hours

Servings: 1

Ingredients:

- Chicken breast (6-lbs., 2.7-kgs)
- The Rub
- Salt – ¼ cup
- Chili powder – 2 tablespoons
- Chinese five-spice – 2 tablespoons
- Brown sugar – 1 ½ cups
- The Smoke
- Preheat the smoker an hour before smoking.
- Add soaked hickory wood chips during the smoking time.
- Black tea – 2 cups

Directions:

1. Place salt, chili powder, Chinese five-spice, and brown sugar in a bowl then stir to combine.
2. Rub the chicken breast with the spice mixture then marinate overnight. Store in the refrigerator to keep it fresh.
3. In the morning, preheat a smoker to 225°F (107°C) with charcoal and hickory wood chips. Prepare indirect heat.

4. Pour black tea into a disposable aluminum pan then place in the smoker.

5. Remove the chicken from the refrigerator then thaw while waiting for the smoker.

6. Once the smoker has reached the desired temperature, place the chicken on the smoker's rack.

7. Smoke the chicken breast for 2 hours then check whether the internal temperature has reached 160°F (71°C).

8. Take the smoked chicken breast out from the smoker and transfer it to a serving dish.

9. Serve and enjoy immediately.

Nutrition: Carbohydrates: 27 g Protein: 19 g Sodium: 65 mg Cholesterol: 49 mg

13. *Sweet Smoked Gingery Lemon Chicken*

Preparation Time: 30 minutes

Cooking Time: 6 Hours

Servings: 1

Ingredients:

- Whole chicken 2 (4-lbs., 1.8-kgs)
- Olive oil – ¼ cup
- The Rub
- Salt – ¼ cup
- Pepper – 2 tablespoons
- Garlic powder – ¼ cup
- The Filling
- Fresh Ginger – 8, 1-inch each
- Cinnamon sticks – 8
- Sliced lemon – ½ cup
- Cloves - 6
- The Smoke
- Preheat the smoker an hour before smoking.
- Add soaked hickory wood chips during the smoking time.

Directions:

1. Preheat a smoker to 225°F (107°C). Use soaked hickory wood chips to make indirect heat.

2. Rub the chicken with salt, pepper, and garlic powder then set aside.

3. Fill the chicken cavities with ginger, cinnamon sticks, cloves, and sliced lemon then brush olive oil all over the chicken.

4. When the smoker is ready, place the whole chicken on the smoker's rack.

5. Smoke the whole chicken for 4 hours then check whether the internal temperature has reached 160°F (71°C).

6. When the chicken is done, remove the smoked chicken from the smoker then let it warm for a few minutes.

7. Serve and enjoy right away or cut into slices.

Nutrition: Carbohydrates: 27 g Protein: 19 g Sodium: 65 mg Cholesterol: 49 mg

BEEF RECIPES

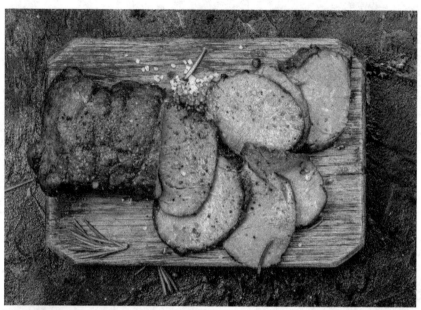

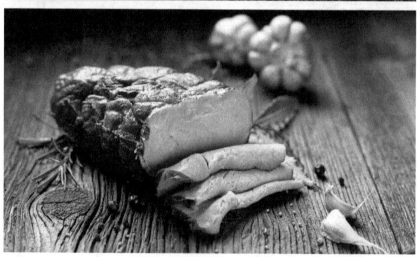

14. Wood Pellet Cocoa Rub Steak

Preparation Time: 20 minutes

Cooking Time: 40 minutes

Servings: 4

Ingredients:

- 4 ribeye steaks
- 2 tablespoons of unsweetened cocoa powder
- 1 tablespoon of dark brown sugar
- 1 tablespoon of smoked paprika
- 1 teaspoon of sea salt to taste
- 1 teaspoon of black pepper
- ½ teaspoon of garlic powder
- ½ teaspoon of onion powder

Directions:

1. Using a large mixing bowl, add in the cocoa powder, brown sugar, paprika, garlic powder, onion powder, and salt to taste then mix properly to combine
2. Rub the steak with about two tablespoons of the spice mixture, coating all sides then let rest for a few minutes.
3. Preheat the Wood Pellet Smoker and Grill to 450 degrees F, place the steak on the grill, and grill for a few minutes on both sides until it is cooked as desired.

---

4. Once cooked, cover the steak in foil and let rest for a few minutes. Serve and enjoy.

Nutrition: Calories: 480 | Fat: 30g | Carbs: 4g | Protein: 40g

15. _Grilled Steak with Mushroom Cream Sauce_

Preparation Time: 25 minutes

Cooking Time: 1 hour and 30 minutes

Servings: 6

Ingredients:

- ½ cup of Dijon mustard
- 2 minced cloves of garlic
- 2 tablespoons of bourbon
- 1 tablespoon of Worcestershire sauce
- 4 beefsteak tenderloin
- 1 tablespoon of peppercorns

Others:

- 1 tablespoon of extra-virgin olive oil
- 1 small and diced onion
- 1 minced clove of garlic
- ½ cup of white wine
- ½ cup of chicken stock
- 16 ounces of sliced mushrooms
- ½ cup of heavy cream
- Salt and pepper to taste

Directions:

1. Using a small mixing bowl, add in the mustard, garlic, bourbon, and Worcestershire sauce then mix properly to combine

2. Place the steak in a Ziploc back, pour in the mustard mixture then shake properly to coat. Let the steak sit for about sixty minutes.

3. Using a small mixing bowl, add in the peppercorns, salt, and pepper to taste then mix to combine.

4. Remove the steak from the Ziploc bag, season the steak with the peppercorn mixture then use clean hands to evenly distribute the seasoning.

5. Preheat the Wood Pellet Smoker and grill to 180 degrees F then close the lid for fifteen minutes.

6. Add the seasoned steak to the grill and smoke for about sixty minutes. Take the steak out of the grill, increase the temperature of the grill to 350 degrees, and grill for 20 to 30 minutes until it attains an internal temperature of 130 degrees F.

7. To make the sauce, place a pan on the pellet grill, add in oil and onions then cook for a few minutes.

8. Cook the garlic for one minute. Add in the mushrooms and cook for a few more minutes.

9. Add in the stock, wine, salt, and pepper to taste, stir to combine then bring to a simmer. Simmer the sauce for 5 to 7 minutes then add in the heavy cream.

10. Stir to combine then serve the steak with the sauce, enjoy.

Nutrition: Calories: 470 | Fat: 25g | Carbs: 10g | Protein: 50g

16. Beef Tenderloin

Preparation Time: 10 minutes

Cooking Time: 1 hour 20 minutes

Servings: 12

Ingredients:

- 1 (5-pound) beef tenderloin, trimmed
- Kosher salt, as required
- ¼ cup olive oil
- Freshly ground black pepper, as required

Directions:

1. With kitchen strings, tie the tenderloin at 7-8 places.
2. Season tenderloin with kosher salt generously.
3. With plastic wrap, cover the tenderloin and keep it aside at room temperature for about 1 hour.
4. Preheat the Z Grills Wood Pellet Grill & Smoker to grill setting to 225-250 degrees F.
5. Coat tenderloin with oil evenly and season with black pepper.
6. Arrange tenderloin onto the grill and cook for about 55-65 minutes.
7. Place cooking grate directly over hot coals and sear tenderloin for about 2 minutes per side.
8. Remove the tenderloin from the grill and place it onto a cutting board for about 10-15 minutes before serving.

9. With a sharp knife, cut the tenderloin into desired-sized slices and serve.

Nutrition: Calories: 425 | Fat: 21g Cholesterol: 170mg | Protein: 55g

17. *Mustard Beef Short Ribs*

Preparation Time: 15 minutes

Cooking Time: 3 hours

Servings: 6

Ingredients:

- For Mustard Sauce:
- 1 cup prepared yellow mustard
- ¼ cup red wine vinegar
- ¼ cup dill pickle juice
- 2 tablespoons soy sauce
- 2 tablespoons Worcestershire sauce
- 1 teaspoon ground ginger
- 1 teaspoon granulated garlic
- For Spice Rub:
- 2 tablespoons salt
- 2 tablespoons freshly ground black pepper
- 1 tablespoon white cane sugar
- 1 tablespoon granulated garlic
- For Ribs:
- 6 (14-ounce) (4-5-inch long) beef short ribs

Directions:

1. Preheat the Z Grills Wood Pellet Grill & Smoker on the smoke setting to 230-250 degrees F, using charcoal.
2. For sauce:
3. In a bowl, mix all ingredients.
4. For rub:
5. In a small bowl, mix all ingredients.
6. Coat the ribs with sauce generously and then sprinkle with spice rub evenly.
7. Place the ribs onto the grill over indirect heat, bone side down. Cook for about 1-1½ hours.
8. Flip the side and cook for about 45 minutes. Repeat.
9. Remove the ribs from the grill and place them onto a cutting board for about 10 minutes before serving.
10. With a sharp knife, cut the ribs into equal-sized individual pieces and serve.

Nutrition: Calories: 867 | Fat: 37g Cholesterol: 361mg | Carbs: 7g | Protein: 117g

LAMB RECIPES

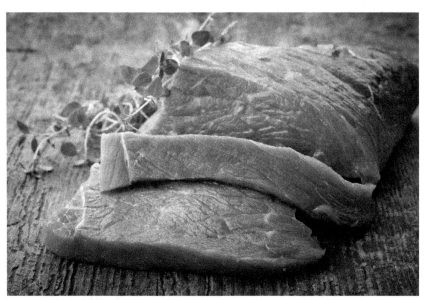

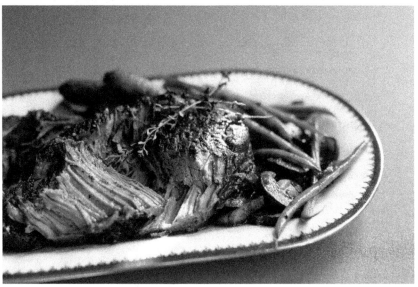

18. *Spicy & Tangy Lamb Shoulder*

Preparation Time; 30 minutes

Cooking Time: 5¾ Hours

Servings: 6

Ingredients:

- 1 (5-lb.) bone-in lamb shoulder, trimmed
- 3-4 tbsp. Moroccan seasoning
- 2 tbsp. olive oil
- 1 C. water
- ¼ C. apple cider vinegar

Directions:

1. Set the temperature of the Grill to 275 degrees F and preheat with a closed lid for 15 minutes, using charcoal.
2. Coat the lamb shoulder with oil evenly and then rub with Moroccan seasoning generously.
3. Place the lamb shoulder onto the grill and cook for about 45 minutes.
4. In a food-safe spray bottle, mix vinegar and water.
5. Spray the lamb shoulder with vinegar mixture evenly.
6. Cook for about 4-5 hours, spraying with vinegar mixture after every 20 minutes.
7. Remove the lamb shoulder from the grill and place onto a cutting board for about 20 minutes before slicing.

8. With a sharp knife, cut the lamb shoulder in desired-sized slices and serve.

Nutrition: Calories per serving: 563; Carbohydrates: 3.1g; Protein: 77.4g; Fat: 25.2g; Sugar: 1.4g; Sodium: 1192mg; Fiber: 0g

19. *Cheesy Lamb Burgers*

Preparation Time: 15 minutes

Cooking Time: 20 Minutes

Servings: 4

Ingredients:

- 2 lb. ground lamb
- 1 C. Parmigiano-Reggiano cheese, grated
- Salt and freshly ground black pepper, to taste

Directions:

1. Set the temperature of the Grill to 425 degrees F and preheat with a closed lid for 15 minutes.
2. In a bowl, add all ingredients and mix well.
3. Make 4 (¾-inch thick) patties from the mixture.
4. With your thumbs, make a shallow but wide depression in each patty.
5. Arrange the patties onto the grill, depression-side down, and cook for about 8 minutes.
6. Flip and cook for about 8-10 minutes.
7. Serve immediately.

Nutrition: Calories per serving: 502; Carbohydrates: 0g; Protein: 71.7g; Fat: 22.6g; Sugar: 0g; Sodium: 331mg; Fiber: 0g

20. Lamb Breast

Preparation Time: 30 minutes

Cooking Time: 2 Hours and 40 Minutes

Servings: 2

Ingredients:

- 1 (2-pound) trimmed bone-in lamb breast
- ½ cup white vinegar
- ¼ cup yellow mustard
- ½ cup BBQ rub

Directions:

1. Preheat the pallet grill to 225 degrees F.
2. Rinse the lamb breast with vinegar evenly.
3. Coat lamb breast with mustard and season with BBQ rub evenly.
4. Arrange lamb breast in pallet grill and cook for about 2-2½ hours.
5. Remove the lamb breast from the pallet grill and transfer onto a cutting board for about 10 minutes before slicing.
6. With a sharp knife, cut the lamb breast in desired-sized slices and serve.

Nutrition: Calories: 877 Cal Fat: 34.5 g Carbohydrates: 2.2 g Protein: 128.7 g Fiber: 0 g

21. *Braised Lamb*

Preparation Time: 30 minutes

Cooking Time: 3 Hours and 20 Minutes

Servings: 4

Ingredients:

- 4 lamb shanks
- Prime rib rub
- 1 cup red wine
- 1 cup beef broth
- 2 sprigs thyme
- 2 sprigs rosemary

Directions:

1. Sprinkle all sides of lamb shanks with prime rib rub.
2. Set temperature of the wood pellet grill to high.
3. Preheat it for 15 minutes while the lid is closed.
4. Add the lamb to the grill and cook for 20 minutes.
5. Transfer the lamb to a Dutch oven.
6. Stir in the rest of the ingredients.
7. Transfer back to the grill.
8. Reduce temperature to 325 degrees F.
9. Braise the lamb for 3 hours.
10. Tips: Let cool before serving.
11. Pour over the sauce.

Nutrition: Calories per serving: 719; Protein: 51.9g; Carbs: 15.4g; Fat: 51g Sugar: 6.9g

22. Grilled Leg Of Lambs Steaks

Preparation Time; 5 minutes

Cooking Time: 10 Minutes

Servings: 4

Ingredients:

- 4 lamb steaks, bone-in
- 1/4 cup olive oil
- 4 garlic cloves, minced
- 1 tbsp. rosemary, freshly chopped
- Salt and black pepper

Directions:

1. Place the lamb in a shallow dish in a single layer. Top with oil, garlic cloves, rosemary, salt, and black pepper then flip the steaks to cover on both sides.
2. Let sit for 30 minutes to marinate.
3. Preheat the wood pellet grill to high and brush the grill grate with oil.
4. Place the lamb steaks on the grill grate and cook until browned and the internal is slightly pink. The internal temperature should be 140 F.
5. Let rest for 5 minutes before serving. Enjoy.

Nutrition: Calories 327, Total Fat 21.9g, Saturated fat 5g, Total Carbs 1.7g, Net Carbs 1.5g, Protein 29.6g, Sugar 0g, Fiber 0.2g, Sodium: 112mg, Potassium 410mg.

PORK RECIPES

23. *Pork Sirloin Tip Roast Three Ways*

Preparation Time: 20 minutes

Cooking Time: 1½ to 3 hours

Servings: 4 to 6

Ingredients:

- Pellet: Apple, Hickory
- Apple-injected Roasted Pork Sirloin Tip Roast
- 1 (1½ to 2 pounds) pork sirloin tip roast
- ¾ cup 100% apple juice
- 2 tablespoons roasted garlic–seasoned extra-virgin olive oil
- 5 tablespoons Pork Dry Rub or a business rub, for example, Plowboys BBQ Bovine Bold

Directions:

1. Dry the roast with a piece of paper
2. Utilize a flavor/marinade injector to infuse all zones of tip roast with the apple juice.
3. Rub the whole roast with olive oil and afterward cover generously with the rub.
4. Utilize 2 silicone nourishment grade cooking groups or butcher's twine to support the roast.

5. Roast the meat until the internal temperature arrives at 145°F, about 1½ hours.

6. Rest the roast under a free foil tent for 15 minutes.

7. Remove the cooking groups or twine and cut the roast contrary to what would be expected.

Nutrition: Calories: 354 kCal   Protein: 22 g   Fat: 30 g

24. Hickory-Smoked Pork Sirloin Tip Roast

Preparation Time: 30 minutes

Cooking Time: 3 hours

Servings: 3

Ingredients:

- 1 (1½ to 2 pounds) pork sirloin tip roast
- 2 tablespoons roasted garlic–seasoned extra-virgin olive oil
- 5 tablespoons Jan's Original Dry Rub, Pork Dry Rub, or your preferred pork rub

Directions:

1. Pat the roast dry with a paper towel.
2. Rub the whole roast with olive oil. Coat the roast with the rub.
3. Support the roast utilizing 2 to 3 silicone nourishment grade cooking groups or butcher's twine to ensure the roast keeps up its shape during cooking.
4. Wrap the tip roast in plastic wrap and refrigerate medium-term.
5. Place the roast directly on the grill grates and smoke the roast until the internal temperature, at the thickest part of the roast, arrives at 145°F, around 3 hours.
6. Rest the roast under a free foil tent for 15 minutes.

7. Remove the cooking groups or twine and cut the roast contrary to what would be expected.

Nutrition: Calories: 276 kCal   Protein: 28 g   Fat: 12 g

25. *Double-Smoked Ham*

Preparation Time: 15 minutes

Cooking Time: 2½ to 3 hours

Servings: 8 to 12

Ingredients:

- Pellet: Apple, Hickory
- 1 (10-pound) applewood-smoked, boneless, wholly cooked, ready-to-eat ham or bone-in smoked ham

Directions:

1. Remove the ham from its bundling and let sit at room temperature for 30 minutes.
2. Arrange the wood pellet smoker-grill for non-direct cooking and preheat to 180°F utilizing apple or hickory pellets relying upon what sort of wood was utilized for the underlying smoking.
3. Place the ham directly on the grill grates and smoke the ham for 1 hour at 180°F.
4. After 60 minutes, increase pit temperature to 350°F.
5. **Cooking Time** the ham until the internal temperature arrives at 140°F, about 1½ to 2 additional hours.
6. Remove the ham and wrap it in foil for 15 minutes before cutting contrary to what would be expected.

Nutrition: Calories: 215 kCal   Protein: 21 g   Fat: 19 g

APPETIZERS AND SIDES

26. *Savory Applesauce on the Grill*

Preparation Time: 0 minutes

Cooking Time: 45 minutes

Servings: 2

Ingredients:

- 1½ pounds whole apples
- Salt

Directions:

1. Start the coals or heat a gas grill for medium direct cooking. Make sure the grates are clean.

2. Put the apples on the grill directly over the fire. Close the lid and cook until the fruit feels soft when gently squeezed with tongs, 10 to 20 minutes total, depending on their size. Transfer to a cutting board and let sit until cool enough to touch.

3. Cut the flesh from around the core of each apple; discard the cores. Put the chunks in a blender or food processor and process until smooth, or put them in a bowl and purée with an immersion blender until as chunky or smooth as you like. Add a generous pinch of salt, then taste and adjust the

seasoning. Serve or refrigerate in an airtight container for up to 3 days.

Nutrition: Calories: 15 Fats: 0 g Cholesterol: 0 mg Carbohydrates: 3 g Fiber: 0 g Sugars: 3 g Proteins: 0 g

27. *Avocado with Lemon*

Preparation Time: 5 minutes

Cooking Time: 20 minutes

Servings: 4

Ingredients:

- 2 ripe avocados
- Good-quality olive oil for brushing
- 1 lemon, halved
- Salt and pepper

Directions:

1. Start the coals or heat a gas grill for medium direct cooking. Make sure the grates are clean.

2. Cut the avocados in half lengthwise. Carefully strike a chef's knife into the pit, then wiggle it a bit to lift and remove it. Insert a spoon underneath the flesh against the skin and run it all the way around to separate the entire half of the avocado. Repeat with the other avocado. Brush with oil, and then squeeze one of the lemon halves over them thoroughly on both sides, so they don't discolor. Cut the other lemon half into 4 wedges.

3. Put the avocados on the grill directly over the fire, cut side down. Close the lid and cook, turning once, until browned in places, 5 to 10 minutes total. Serve the halved avocados as is,

or slice and fan them for a prettier presentation. Sprinkle with salt and pepper and garnish with lemon wedges.

Nutrition: Calories: 50.3 Fats: 4.6 g Cholesterol: 0 mg Carbohydrates: 2.8 g Fiber: 1.7 g Sugars: 0.2 g Proteins: 0.6 g

28. Simplest Grilled Asparagus

Preparation Time: 0 minutes

Cooking Time: 25 minutes

Servings: 4

Ingredients:

- 1½–2 pounds asparagus
- 1–2 tablespoons good-quality olive oil or melted butter
- Salt

Directions:

1. Start the coals or heat a gas grill for direct hot cooking. Make sure the grates are clean.
2. Cut the tough bottoms from the asparagus. If they're thick, trim the ends with a vegetable peeler. Toss with the oil and sprinkle with salt.
3. Put the asparagus on the grill directly over the fire, perpendicular to the grates, so they don't fall through. Close the lid and cook, turning once, until the thick part of the stalks can barely be pierced with a skewer or thin knife, 5 to 10 minutes total. Transfer to a platter and serve.

Nutrition: Calories: 225 Fats: 20.6 g Cholesterol: 0 mg Carbohydrates: 9.1 g Fiber: 4.2 g Sugars: 0 g Proteins: 4.6 g

29. *Beets and Greens with Lemon-Dill Vinaigrette*

Preparation Time: 0 minutes

Cooking Time: 1 hour

Servings: 4

Ingredients:

- 1½ pounds small beets, with fresh-looking greens still attached if possible
- ½ cup plus 2 tablespoons good-quality olive oil
- Salt and pepper
- 3 tablespoons fresh lemon juice
- 2 tablespoons minced fresh dill

Directions:

1. Start the coals or heat a gas grill for medium to medium-low direct cooking. Make sure the grates are clean.
2. Cut the greens off the beets. Throw away any wilted or discolored leaves; rinse the remainder thoroughly to remove any grit and drain. Trim the root ends of the beets and scrub well under running water. Pat the leaves and beets dry. Toss the beets with 2 tablespoons of oil and a sprinkle of salt until evenly coated.
3. Put the beets on the grill directly over the fire. (No need to wash the bowl.) Close the lid and cook, turning them every 5 to 10 minutes, until a knife inserted in the center goes through

with no resistance, 30 to 40 minutes total. Transfer to a plate and let sit until cool enough to handle.

4. Toss the beet greens in the reserved bowl to coat in oil. Put the greens on the grill directly over the fire. Close the lid and cook, tossing once or twice, until they're bright green and browned in spots, 2 to 5 minutes total. Keep a close eye on them; if they're on too long, they'll crisp up to the point where they'll shatter. Transfer to a plate.

5. Put the remaining ½ cup oil and the lemon juice in a serving bowl and whisk until thickened. Stir in the dill and some salt and pepper. Peel the skin from the beets and cut into halves or quarters. Cut the stems from the leaves in 1-inch lengths; cut the leaves across into ribbons. Put the beets, leaves, and stems in the bowl and toss with the vinaigrette until coated. Serve warm or at room temperature. Or makeup to several hours ahead, cover, and refrigerate to serve chilled.

Nutrition: Calories: 73 Fats: 3.8 g Cholesterol: 0 mg Carbohydrates: 9.6 g Fiber: 3.6 g Sugars: 2 g Proteins: 2.2 g

VEGETARIAN RECIPES

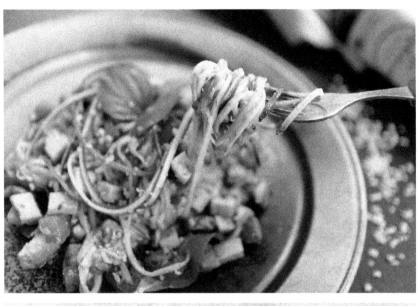

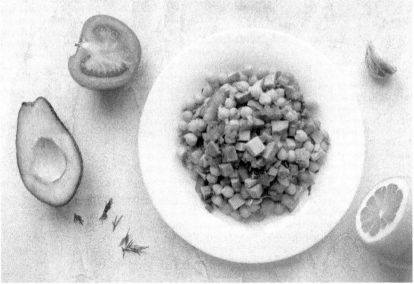

30. <u>Mushrooms Stuffed with Crab Meat</u>

Preparation Time: 20 Minutes

Cooking Time: 45 Minutes

Servings: 6

Ingredients:

- 6 medium-sized Portobello mushrooms
- Extra virgin olive oil
- 1/3 Grated parmesan cheese cup
- Club Beat Staffing:
- 8 ounces fresh crab meat or canned or imitation crab meat
- 2 tablespoons extra virgin olive oil
- 1/3 Chopped celery
- Chopped red peppers
- ½ cup chopped green onion
- ½ cup Italian bread crumbs

Directions:

1. Clean up the mushroom cap with a damp paper towel. Cut off the stem and save it.
2. Remove the brown gills from the bottom of the mushroom cap with a spoon and discard.
3. Prepare crab meat stuffing. If you are a fan of using canned crab meat, drain, rinse, and remove shellfish.

4. Put the crab mixture in each mushroom cap and make a mound in the center.

5. Sprinkle extra virgin olive oil and sprinkle parmesan cheese on each stuffed mushroom cap. Put the mushrooms in a 10 x 15-inch baking dish.

6. Use the pellets to set the wood pellet smoker and grill to indirect heating and preheat to 375 ° F.

7. Bake for 30-45 minutes until the filling becomes hot (165 degrees Fahrenheit as measured by an instant-read digital thermometer). The mushrooms begin to release juice.

Nutrition: Calories: 160 Carbs: 14g Fat: 8g Protein: 10g

31. *Apple Wood Smoked Cheese*

Preparation Time: 1 Hour and 15 Minutes

Cooking Time: 2 Hours

Servings: 6

Ingredients:

- Gouda

- Sharp cheddar

- Very sharp 3-year cheddar

- Monterey Jack

- Pepper jack

- Swiss

Directions:

1. According to the cheese block's shape, cut the cheese block into an easy-to-handle size (approximately 4 x 4-inch block) to promote smoke penetration.

2. Leave the cheese on the counter for one hour to form a very thin skin or crust, which acts as a heat barrier, but allows smoke to penetrate.

3. Configure the wood pellet smoking grill for indirect heating and install a cold smokebox to prepare for cold smoke. Ensure that the louvers on the smoking box are fully open to allow moisture to escape from the box.

4. Preheat the wood pellet smoker and grill to 180 ° F or use apple pellets and smoke settings, if any, to get a milder smoke flavor.

5. Place the cheese on a Teflon-coated fiberglass non-stick grill mat and let cool for 2 hours.

6. Remove the smoked cheese and cool for 1 hour on the counter using a cooling rack.

7. After labeling the smoked cheese with a vacuum seal, refrigerate for 2 weeks or more. Smoke will permeate and the cheese flavor will become milder.

Nutrition: Calories: 102 Carbs: 0g Fat: 9 Protein: 6g

32. Smoked Guacamole

Preparation Time: 15 Minutes

Cooking Time: 30 Minutes

Servings: 8

Ingredients:

- 1/4 cup chopped Cilantro
- 7 Avocados, peeled and seeded
- ¼ cup chopped Onion, red
- ¼ cup chopped tomato
- 3 ears corn
- 1 teaspoon of Chile Powder
- 1 teaspoon of Cumin
- 2 tablespoons of Lime juice
- 1 tablespoon minced Garlic
- 1 Chile, poblano
- Black pepper and salt to taste

Directions:

1. Preheat the grill to 180F with a closed lid.
2. Smoke the avocado for 10 min.
3. Set the avocados aside and increase the temperature of the girl to high.
4. Once heated grill the corn and chili. Roast for 20 minutes.

5. Cut the corn. Set aside. Place the chili in a bowl. Cover it with a wrapper and let it sit for about 10 minutes. Peel the chili and dice. Add it to the kernels.

6. In a bowl mash the avocados, leave few chunks. Add the remaining ingredients and mix.

7. Serve right away because it is best eaten fresh. Enjoy!

Nutrition: Calories: 51 Protein: 1g Carbs: 3g Fat: 4.5g

33. Corn Salsa

Preparation Time: 10 Minutes

Cooking Time: 15 Minutes

Servings: 4

Ingredients:

- 4 Ears Corn, large with the husk on

- 4 Tomatoes (Roma) diced and seeded

- 1 teaspoon of onion powder

- 1 teaspoon of Garlic powder

- 1 Onion, diced

- 1/2 cup chopped Cilantro

- Black pepper and salt to taste

- 1 lime, the juice

- 1 grille jalapeno, diced

Directions:

1. Preheat the grill to 450F.

2. Place the ears corn on the grate and cook until charred. Remove husk. Cut into kernels.

3. Combine all ingredients, plus the corn, and mix well. Refrigerate before serving.

Nutrition: Calories: 120 Protein: 2g Carbs: 4g Fat: 1g

GAME AND ORIGINAL RECIPES

34. *Spicy Barbecue Pecans*

Preparation Time: 15 Minutes

Cooking Time: 1 Hour

Servings: 2

Ingredients:

- 2 ½ t. garlic powder
- 16 ounces raw pecan halves
- One t. onion powder
- One t. pepper
- Two t. salt
- One t. dried thyme
- Butter, for greasing
- 3 T. melted butter

Directions:

1. Add wood pellets to your smoker and follow your cooker's startup method.
2. Preheat your smoker, with your lid closed, until it reaches 225.

3. Cover and smoke for an hour, flipping the nuts one. Make sure the nuts are toasted and heated. They should be removed from the grill.

4. Set aside to cool and dry.

Nutrition: Calories: 150 Carbs: 16g Fat: 9g Protein: 1g

35. *Feta Cheese Stuffed Meatballs*

Preparation Time: 12 Minutes

Cooking Time: 35 Minutes

Servings: 6

Ingredients:

- Pepper
- Salt
- ¾ c. Feta cheese
- ½ t. thyme
- Two t. chopped oregano
- Zest of one lemon
- One-pound ground pork
- One-pound ground beef
- One T. olive oil

Directions:

1. Place the pepper, salt, thyme, oregano, olive oil, lemon zest, and ground meats into a large bowl.
2. Combine the ingredients thoroughly using your hands.
3. Cut the Feta into little cubes and begin making the meatballs. Take a half tablespoon of the meat mixture and roll it around a piece of cheese. Continue until all meat has been used.

4. Add wood pellets to your smoker and follow your cooker's startup procedure.

5. Preheat your smoker, with your lid closed, until it reaches 350.

6. Brush the meatballs with more olive oil and put them onto the grill. Grill for ten minutes until browned.

Nutrition: Calories: 390 Carbs: 8g Fat: 31g Protein: 20g

36. *Butternut Squash*

Preparation Time: 30 Minutes

Cooking Time: 2 Hours

Servings: 4-6

Ingredients:

- Brown sugar
- Maple syrup
- 6 T. butter
- Butternut squash

Directions:

1. Add wood pellets to your smoker and follow your cooker's startup procedure. Preheat your smoke, with your lid closed, until it reaches 300.
2. Place each half of the squash onto aluminum foil.
3. Increase temperature to 400 and place onto the grill for another 35 minutes.
4. Carefully unwrap each half, making sure to reserve juices in the bottom. Place onto serving platter and drizzle juices over each half. Use a spoon to scoop out and enjoy.

Nutrition: Calories: 82 Carbs: 22g Fat: 0g Protein: 2g

SNACKS

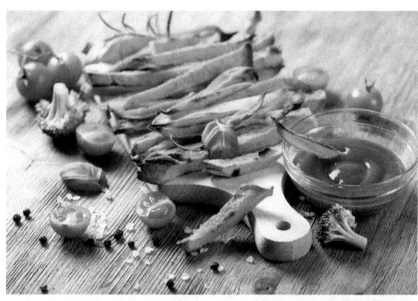

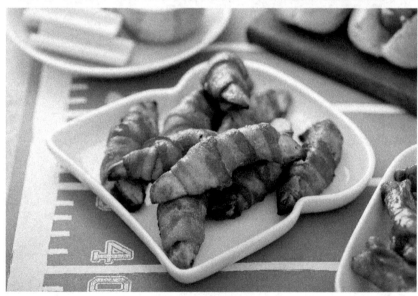

37. *Grilled Watermelon*

Preparation Time: 5 minutes

Cooking Time: 2 minutes

Servings: 2-3

Ingredients:

- 6 watermelon slices, each measuring 3 inches across and 1-inch thick
- 2 tablespoons honey

Directions:

1. Put the grill grate inside the hood and close the unit.
2. Set temperature to the max and set the timer to 2 minutes.
3. Stop the unit as it is preheated.
4. Now brush the watermelon slices with honey.
5. Grease the grill grate with oil spray.
6. Place the watermelon slices on the grill grate.
7. Close the hood and grill for 2 minutes without flipping it.
8. Once done, take out watermelon slices and serve them immediately.

Nutrition: Calories: 322 | Total Fat: 1.1g | Saturated Fat: 0.6g Cholesterol: 0mg | Sodium: 12mg

Total Carbohydrate: 81.8g Dietary Fiber: 3.4g Total Sugars: 69.9g | Protein: 5.1g